Navigating Hypertension Tips & Tools for Patients & Families

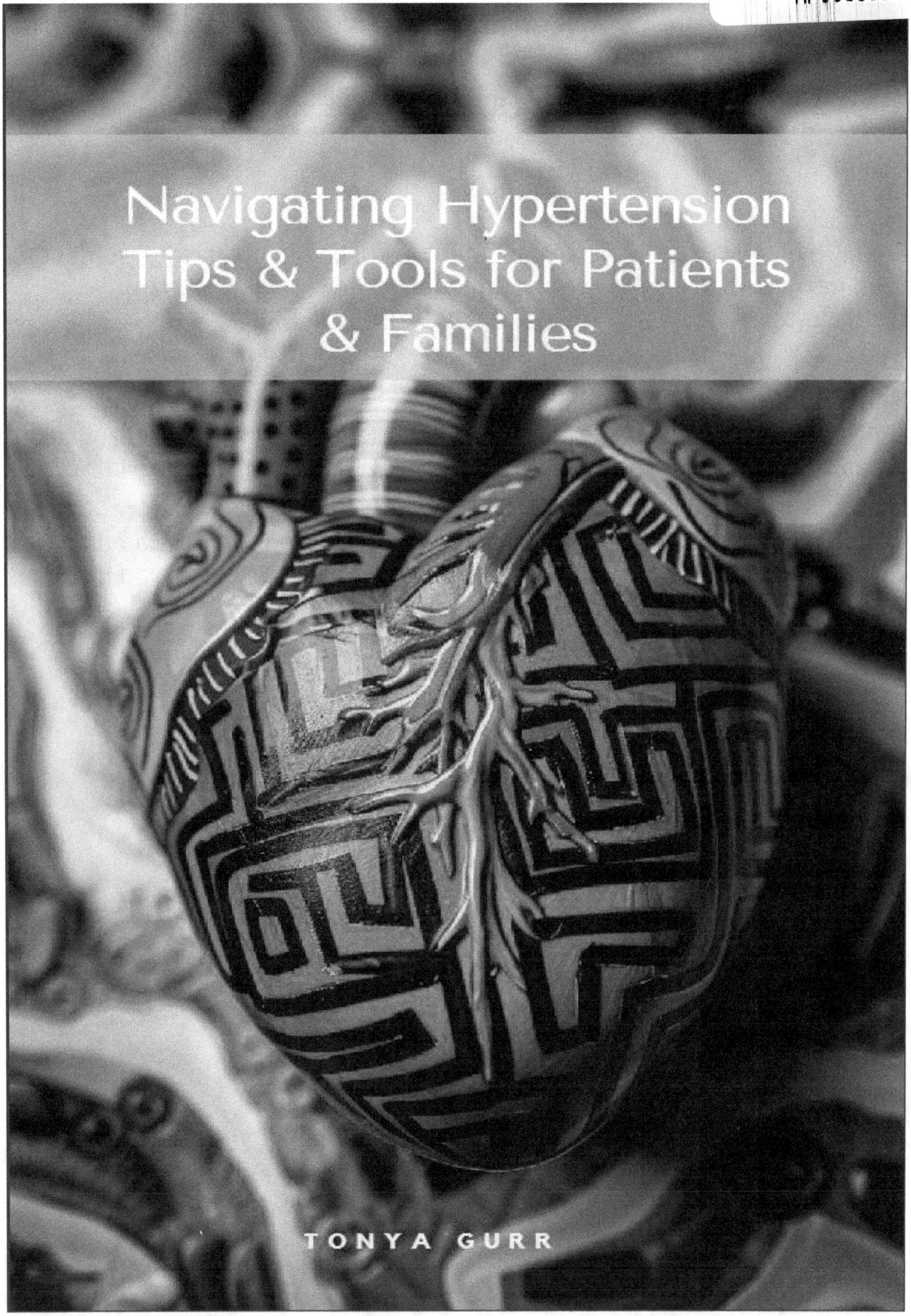

TONYA GURR

Dedication

To my mother, Ora Lee my daughter Mary, cherished family, steadfast friends, and the remarkable souls I've encountered on life's winding journey,

Your unwavering support, love, and shared moments have woven the fabric of my existence. Each fleeting or enduring encounter has left an indelible mark on my heart.

In gratitude, I dedicate this book to you—the silent encouragers, the laughter sharers, and the compassionate listeners. May its pages resonate with your stories and inspire kindness in your every step.

Remember Charles H. Kraft's timeless wisdom: "Spread kindness around like confetti." Let our lives be a celebration of compassion, empathy, and love.

With heartfelt appreciation,

Tonya

P.S. I thank Ine Velaers for the generation of the Cover Art, and CDW for always believing!

Table of Contents

Introduction

Chapter 1   Understanding Hypertension

Chapter 2   Diagnosing Hypertension

Chapter 3   Managing Hypertension Through Lifestyle Modification

Chapter 4   Medications for Hypertension

Chapter 5   Monitoring Your Blood Pressure

Chapter 6   Support for Patients & Families

Chapter 7   Navigating Hypertension in Special Situations

Chapter 8   Resources for Managing Hypertension

Chapter 9   Planning for the Future

Chapter 10   Conclusion

References   Identified by Chapter

Introduction

My Journey with Hypertension

Hypertension, commonly known as high blood pressure, is a condition that affects millions of people worldwide, and I am one of them. My name is Tonya, I am a military veteran approaching the age of 60. Despite knowing that I had high blood pressure, I, like many others, believed I could manage it on my own. I thought I could beat it through sheer willpower and minor lifestyle adjustments. However, my story took a dramatic turn when I experienced a hypertensive crisis that changed my perspective on the severity of this condition.

It was a day like any other until I felt a sudden and overwhelming sensation as if my body was on the verge of exploding. My blood pressure had skyrocketed to a dangerous 218/166. In those frightening moments, I realized the true gravity of uncontrolled hypertension. The paramedics were called, and their prompt intervention likely saved my life. This experience was a wake-up call, a stark reminder that hypertension is not something to be taken lightly or managed alone without proper medical guidance.

The Purpose of This Book

This book, "Navigating Hypertension: Tips and Tools for Patients and Families," is born out of my personal experience and the need to share vital information with others who may be facing similar challenges. Hypertension is often referred to as the "silent killer" because it can cause significant damage to the body without obvious symptoms. My goal is to provide a comprehensive resource that covers all aspects of hypertension management, from understanding the condition to effectively controlling it through lifestyle modifications, medications, and ongoing monitoring.

Why This Book Matters

Hypertension is a complex condition influenced by various factors, including genetics, lifestyle, and environmental influences. Effective management requires a multifaceted approach, encompassing education, support, and the right tools. This book is designed to empower patients and their families with knowledge and strategies to take control of their health.

Throughout the chapters, you will find detailed information on the following topics:

- **Understanding Hypertension:** An overview of the condition, its types, and its global impact.
- **Diagnosing Hypertension:** Methods and criteria for accurate diagnosis.
- **Managing Hypertension Through Lifestyle Modifications:** Practical advice on diet, exercise, stress management, and more.
- **Medications for Hypertension:** An in-depth look at the different classes of antihypertensive drugs, their mechanisms, and managing side effects.
- **Monitoring Your Blood Pressure:** Techniques and tools for effective self-monitoring.
- **Support for Patients and Families:** The critical role of family and caregivers, education strategies, and support resources.
- **Navigating Hypertension in Special Situations:** Tailored approaches for managing hypertension in pregnancy, older adults, and children.
- **Resources for Managing Hypertension:** Technological tools, educational materials, and community resources.
- **Planning for the Future:** Setting goals, regular check-ups, and long-term management strategies.

A Call to Action

Hypertension management is not just about taking medications; it's about adopting a holistic approach to health. This book aims to serve as a guide for patients and their families, offering practical tips and tools to navigate the complexities of hypertension. By taking proactive steps, staying informed, and seeking support, it is possible to live a healthy and fulfilling life despite the challenges posed by high blood pressure.

My journey with hypertension has been a humbling experience, and I hope that sharing it will inspire others to take their health seriously. Whether you are newly diagnosed or have been living with hypertension for years, this book is for you. Let's embark on this journey together, towards better health and a better future.

Chapter 1: Understanding Hypertension

1.1 Definition and Epidemiology

1.1.1 Definition

Hypertension, or high blood pressure, is a condition in which the force exerted by the blood against the walls of the blood vessels is consistently elevated. This condition can lead to significant health problems if left unmanaged. Blood pressure is determined by the amount of blood your heart pumps and the resistance to blood flow in your arteries. The more blood your heart pumps and the narrowing of your arteries, the higher your blood pressure. Hypertension is typically diagnosed based on persistent blood pressure readings above 140/90 mm Hg, though recent guidelines suggest 130/80 mm Hg as the threshold for diagnosis.

1.1.2 Types of Hypertensions

- **Primary (Essential) Hypertension:** The most common type accounts for about 90-95% of cases. It develops gradually over many years and has no identifiable cause but is linked to genetic factors, diet, and lifestyle.
- **Secondary Hypertension:** This type accounts for about 5-10% of cases and is caused by an underlying condition, such as kidney disease, hormonal disorders, or the use of certain medications. It tends to appear suddenly and causes higher blood pressure than primary hypertension.

1.1.3 Global Epidemiology

Hypertension is a major global public health issue affecting over 1.4 billion people worldwide. Its prevalence varies significantly across different regions and populations. In high-income countries, the prevalence of hypertension has stabilized or decreased, likely due to improved healthcare and public health interventions. In contrast, low- and middle-income countries have seen a rise in hypertension prevalence due to urbanization, lifestyle changes, and inadequate healthcare infrastructure.

1.1.4 Risk Factors

Several factors increase the risk of developing hypertension, including:

- **Age:** Risk increases with age, particularly after 45 for men and 55 for women.
- **Race:** Hypertension is more common and often more severe in African American adults.
- **Family History:** A family history of hypertension increases risk.
- **Lifestyle Factors:** Poor diet (high in sodium, low in potassium), physical inactivity, excessive alcohol consumption, and smoking.
- **Obesity:** Excess weight is a significant risk factor for hypertension.
- **Stress:** Chronic stress may contribute to high blood pressure.

1.1.5 Demographic Groups Most Affected

Hypertension disproportionately affects certain demographic groups:

- **Older Adults:** Due to natural aging processes and increased arterial stiffness.
- **Ethnic Minorities:** African Americans have higher rates of hypertension and related complications.
- **Lower Socioeconomic Status:** Associated with higher prevalence due to factors such as limited access to healthcare, unhealthy diets, and higher stress levels.

1.2 Pathophysiology

1.2.1 Autonomic Nervous System

The autonomic nervous system (ANS) plays a critical role in regulating blood pressure. It consists of the sympathetic and parasympathetic nervous systems. The sympathetic nervous system (SNS) increases heart rate and constricts blood vessels, raising blood pressure, while the parasympathetic nervous system (PNS) has the opposite effect. In hypertension, there is often increased SNS activity and decreased PNS activity, leading to sustained high blood pressure.

1.2.2 Renal Function

The kidneys help regulate blood pressure by controlling fluid balance and secreting hormones such as renin, which activates the renin-angiotensin-aldosterone system (RAAS). Dysfunction in renal sodium handling can lead to volume overload and hypertension. Additionally, kidney disease can cause secondary hypertension due to impaired renal function and increased renin release.

1.2.3 Renin-Angiotensin-Aldosterone System (RAAS)

RAAS is a hormone system that regulates blood pressure and fluid balance. When blood volume is low, the kidneys release renin, which converts angiotensinogen to angiotensin I. Angiotensin I is then converted to angiotensin II, a potent vasoconstrictor that increases blood pressure by narrowing blood vessels and stimulating aldosterone release from the adrenal glands. Aldosterone promotes sodium and water retention, further increasing blood volume and pressure. Dysregulation of RAAS can contribute to the development and maintenance of hypertension.

1.2.4 Genetic Factors

Genetics plays a significant role in hypertension, with several genes implicated in blood pressure regulation. A family history of hypertension is a strong risk factor, and genetic studies have identified multiple genetic variants associated with increased risk.

1.2.5 Environmental and Behavioral Factors

- **Diet:** High sodium or low potassium intake, and diets high in fat and sugar may contribute to hypertension.
- **Physical Activity:** A sedentary lifestyle is associated with higher risk.
- **Alcohol and Tobacco Use:** Both can increase blood pressure through various mechanisms, including vasoconstriction and increased SNS activity.
- **Stress:** Chronic stress can lead to persistent increases in blood pressure.

1.3 Complications

1.3.1 Cardiovascular Disease

Hypertension is a major risk factor for cardiovascular diseases, including coronary artery disease, heart failure, and arrhythmias. High blood pressure causes damage to the blood vessels, leading to atherosclerosis, which can result in heart attacks and strokes.

1.3.2 Stroke

Uncontrolled hypertension can cause both ischemic and hemorrhagic strokes. High blood pressure damages the blood vessels in the brain, leading to an increased risk of clot formation (ischemic stroke) or vessel rupture (hemorrhagic stroke).

1.3.3 Kidney Disease

Hypertension can damage the blood vessels in the kidneys, impairing their ability to filter waste from the blood. This can lead to chronic kidney disease and, eventually, kidney failure, necessitating dialysis or kidney transplantation.

1.3.4 Vision Loss

High blood pressure can damage the blood vessels in the retina, leading to hypertensive retinopathy. This condition can cause vision problems and, in severe cases, complete vision loss.

1.3.5 Other Complications

Hypertension can also lead to other complications, including:

- **Peripheral Artery Disease**: Reduced blood flow to the limbs, causing pain and mobility issues.
- **Cognitive Impairment and Dementia**: Chronic hypertension is linked to cognitive decline and increased risk of dementia, possibly due to small vessel disease in the brain.
- **Aneurysms**: High blood pressure can cause blood vessels to weaken and bulge, forming aneurysms that can rupture and cause life-threatening bleeding.

Understanding these complexities of hypertension is crucial for effective management and prevention strategies, ultimately reducing the burden of this widespread condition on individuals and healthcare systems.

Chapter 2: Diagnosing Hypertension

2.1 Blood Pressure Measurement Techniques

2.1.1 Office Measurements

Blood pressure (BP) measurement in a clinical setting is the most traditional method. This involves using a sphygmomanometer and a stethoscope or an automated BP monitor. Proper technique is critical for accuracy:

- **Preparation:** Patients should be seated comfortably with their back supported, legs uncrossed, and one arm at heart level. They should rest for at least 5 minutes before the measurement.
- **Procedure:** The cuff should be placed on bare skin, not over clothing, and fit properly (the bladder should cover 80% of the arm circumference). Measurements should be taken in both arms initially, and the higher reading should be used for subsequent measurements.
- **Repeated Readings:** At least two readings, 1-2 minutes apart, should be taken and averaged. Additional measurements may be required if there is a significant difference between the first and second readings.

2.1.2 Home Blood Pressure Monitoring

Home blood pressure monitoring (HBPM) is increasingly recommended for diagnosing and managing hypertension. It provides a more accurate reflection of a person's BP in their usual environment and can help identify white-coat hypertension (elevated BP in clinical settings but normal at home) and masked hypertension (normal BP in clinical settings but elevated at home).

- **Equipment:** Use validated and properly calibrated automated devices.
- **Procedure:** Patients should measure BP at the same times each day, usually in the morning and evening, after sitting quietly for at least 5 minutes. They should take at least two readings each time, 1 minute apart, and record the readings.
- **Advantages:** HBPM can enhance patient involvement in their care and improve treatment adherence.

2.1.3 Ambulatory Blood Pressure Monitoring

Ambulatory blood pressure monitoring (ABPM) involves wearing a portable BP monitor that takes readings at regular intervals (typically every 15-30 minutes during the day and every 30-60 minutes at night) over 24 hours. ABPM is considered the gold standard for BP measurement because it provides a comprehensive profile of BP changes throughout the day and night.

- **Procedure:** The monitor is worn on a belt with the cuff placed on the non-dominant arm. Patients should carry on with their usual daily activities but avoid vigorous exercise.
- **Advantages:** ABPM can detect white-coat and masked hypertension, provides information on nocturnal BP patterns (dipping vs. non-dipping), and offer insights into BP variability.
- **Indications:** ABPM is particularly useful for diagnosing white-coat hypertension, resistant hypertension, and episodic hypertension, and for evaluating the effectiveness of antihypertensive therapy.

2.2 Diagnostic Criteria

2.2.1 American Heart Association (AHA) Guidelines

The AHA defines hypertension based on BP readings obtained through proper measurement techniques. The categories are:

- **Normal:** Systolic BP <120 mm Hg and diastolic BP <80 mm Hg.
- **Elevated:** Systolic BP 120-129 mm Hg and diastolic BP <80 mm Hg.
- **Hypertension Stage 1:** Systolic BP 130-139 mm Hg or diastolic BP 80-89 mm Hg.
- **Hypertension Stage 2:** Systolic BP ≥140 mm Hg or diastolic BP ≥90 mm Hg.
- **Hypertensive Crisis:** Systolic BP >180 mm Hg and/or diastolic BP >120 mm Hg, requiring immediate medical attention.

2.2.2 World Health Organization (WHO) Guidelines

The WHO's criteria for hypertension are similar but may vary slightly based on regional adaptations. Generally, the categories include:

- **Optimal BP:** Systolic BP <120 mm Hg and diastolic BP <80 mm Hg.
- **Normal BP:** Systolic BP 120-129 mm Hg and diastolic BP 80-84 mm Hg.
- **High-Normal BP:** Systolic BP 130-139 mm Hg and diastolic BP 85-89 mm Hg.
- **Hypertension:** Systolic BP ≥140 mm Hg and/or diastolic BP ≥90 mm Hg.

- **Grade 1 Hypertension:** Systolic BP 140-159 mm Hg and/or diastolic BP 90-99 mm Hg.
- **Grade 2 Hypertension:** Systolic BP 160-179 mm Hg and/or diastolic BP 100-109 mm Hg.
- **Grade 3 Hypertension:** Systolic BP ≥180 mm Hg and/or diastolic BP ≥110 mm Hg.

2.3 Secondary Hypertension Screening

2.3.1 Importance of Identifying Secondary Causes

Secondary hypertension is hypertension with an identifiable and potentially treatable cause. It accounts for about 5-10% of hypertension cases. Identifying secondary causes is crucial because treating the underlying condition can resolve or significantly improve hypertension.

2.3.2 Common Causes and Diagnostic Tests

- **Renal Artery Stenosis:** A narrowing of the arteries that supply the kidneys, often due to atherosclerosis or fibromuscular dysplasia. Diagnosis can involve Doppler ultrasound, CT angiography, or MR angiography.
- **Primary Aldosteronism:** An overproduction of aldosterone by the adrenal glands will lead to sodium retention and potassium loss. Screening involves measuring plasma aldosterone concentration and plasma renin activity.
- **Cushing's Syndrome:** Excess cortisol production by the adrenal glands. Diagnostic tests include a 24-hour urinary-free cortisol test, low-dose dexamethasone suppression test, and late-night salivary cortisol test.
- **Pheochromocytoma:** A rare tumor of the adrenal gland that secretes catecholamines, causing episodic hypertension. Diagnosis involves measuring plasma or urinary metanephrines and catecholamines.
- **Coarctation of the Aorta:** A congenital narrowing of the aorta that can cause high blood pressure in the upper body. Diagnosis is confirmed with imaging studies like echocardiography, MRI, or CT angiography.
- **Thyroid Disorders:** Both hyperthyroidism and hypothyroidism can cause hypertension. Screening includes measuring thyroid-stimulating hormone (TSH) and thyroid hormone levels (T3 and T4).

2.3.3 Other Considerations

- **Medication-Induced Hypertension:** Certain medications, such as oral contraceptives, nonsteroidal anti-inflammatory drugs (NSAIDs), and steroids, can raise blood pressure. A thorough medication history is essential.
- **Obstructive Sleep Apnea (OSA):** OSA is linked to resistant hypertension. Screening includes questionnaires and overnight polysomnography.

By following these detailed approaches to diagnosing hypertension, healthcare providers can ensure accurate diagnosis and effective management of both primary and secondary hypertension, ultimately improving patient outcomes.

Chapter 3: Managing Hypertension Through Lifestyle Modifications

3.1 Dietary Interventions

3.1.1 DASH Diet

The Dietary Approaches to Stop Hypertension (DASH) diet is a well-researched and effective dietary plan designed specifically to help lower blood pressure. Key components of the DASH diet include:

- **High in Fruits and Vegetables**: Rich in fiber, potassium, and magnesium, which are beneficial for lowering blood pressure.
- **Low in Saturated Fat and Cholesterol**: Emphasizes lean meats, poultry, fish, and nuts while reducing the intake of red meat, sweets, and sugary beverages.
- **Whole Grains**: Encourages consumption of whole grains over refined grains.
- **Low-Fat Dairy**: Includes low-fat or fat-free dairy products to reduce saturated fat intake.

Clinical trials have shown that the DASH diet can significantly lower systolic and diastolic blood pressure in individuals with hypertension. For example, the original DASH study demonstrated reductions in blood pressure within just two weeks of following the diet.

3.1.2 Sodium Reduction

Excessive sodium intake is a major contributor to hypertension. Reducing sodium intake can help lower blood pressure and improve heart health. Recommendations include:

- **Limit Daily Sodium Intake**: The American Heart Association (AHA) recommends no more than 2,300 milligrams per day, with an ideal limit of 1,500 milligrams per day for most adults.
- **Avoid Processed Foods**: Processed and restaurant foods are typically high in sodium. Opt for fresh, home-cooked meals where sodium levels can be controlled.
- **Read Labels**: Check food labels for sodium content and choose lower-sodium options.

3.1.3 Potassium, Magnesium, and Calcium

These minerals play crucial roles in blood pressure regulation:

- **Potassium:** Helps balance sodium levels in the body. Foods rich in potassium include bananas, oranges, potatoes, and spinach.
- **Magnesium:** Helps regulate blood pressure by relaxing blood vessels. Sources include whole grains, green leafy vegetables, nuts, and seeds.
- **Calcium:** Essential for vascular contraction and vasodilation. Dairy products, fortified plant-based milks, and leafy greens are good sources.

Evidence from clinical trials supports the inclusion of these minerals in the diet for blood pressure management. For instance, increased potassium intake is associated with lower blood pressure, especially when coupled with reduced sodium intake.

3.2 Physical Activity

3.2.1 Aerobic Exercise

Regular aerobic exercise is one of the most effective lifestyle interventions for lowering blood pressure. Recommendations include:

- **Frequency:** At least 150 minutes of moderate-intensity aerobic exercise per week, such as brisk walking, jogging, or cycling.
- **Intensity:** Moderate to vigorous intensity, where moderate intensity is defined as 50-70% of maximum heart rate and vigorous intensity as 70-85%.

3.2.2 Resistance Training

Resistance training also contributes to blood pressure management and overall cardiovascular health:

- **Frequency:** At least two days per week.
- **Exercises:** Focus on major muscle groups using free weights, resistance bands, or bodyweight exercises.

3.2.3 Flexibility and Balance Exercises

While not directly affecting blood pressure, flexibility and balance exercises improve overall fitness and can aid in the prevention of falls, particularly in older adults:

- **Examples:** Yoga, Pilates, and stretching routines.

Clinical evidence suggests that a combination of aerobic and resistance training provides the best outcomes for blood pressure reduction.

3.3 Weight Management

3.3.1 Impact of Obesity on Hypertension

Obesity is a significant risk factor for hypertension due to factors such as increased blood volume, elevated sympathetic nervous system activity, and insulin resistance. Managing weight is critical for controlling blood pressure.

3.3.2 Strategies for Weight Management

- **Dietary Changes:** Adopting a balanced diet, such as the DASH diet or a Mediterranean diet, which emphasizes whole foods, healthy fats, and lean proteins.
- **Physical Activity:** Regular exercise will burn calories and build muscle, which increases metabolic rate.
- **Behavioral Changes:** Techniques such as goal setting, self-monitoring, and seeking support from healthcare providers or support groups.

Clinical studies show that even modest weight loss (5-10% of body weight) reduces blood pressure significantly.

3.4 Stress Management

3.4.1 Mindfulness and Meditation

Mindfulness practices and meditation techniques help reduce stress and lower blood pressure. Techniques include:

- **Mindfulness-Based Stress Reduction (MBSR):** A structured program incorporates mindfulness meditation and yoga.
- **Transcendental Meditation:** A form of silent mantra meditation.

3.4.2 Cognitive-Behavioral Therapy (CBT)

CBT helps individuals manage stress by changing negative thought patterns and behaviors. It is an effective therapy for reducing stress and improving mental health, which can in turn lower blood pressure.

3.4.3 Other Stress Reduction Techniques

- **Deep Breathing Exercises:** Simple breathing techniques that promote relaxation.
- **Progressive Muscle Relaxation:** A method of tensing and relaxing different muscle groups to reduce physical tension.

Research supports the effectiveness of these techniques in reducing both psychological stress and blood pressure.

3.5 Alcohol and Tobacco Use

3.5.1 Effects of Alcohol on Blood Pressure

Excessive alcohol consumption is linked to elevated blood pressure and increased risk of hypertension. Recommendations include:

- **Moderate Consumption:** Up to one drink per day for women and up to two drinks per day for men.
- **Alcohol Reduction Programs:** Structured programs and counseling can help individuals reduce their alcohol intake.

3.5.2 Effects of Tobacco on Blood Pressure

Smoking increases blood pressure and contributes to the development of hypertension through vasoconstriction and arterial damage. Strategies for cessation include:

- **Behavioral Therapy:** Counseling and support groups.
- **Pharmacotherapy:** Nicotine replacement therapy (patches, gum, lozenges), and medications such as bupropion and varenicline.
- **Lifestyle Changes:** Adopting healthier habits to replace smoking triggers.

Evidence shows that reducing alcohol intake and quitting smoking can lead to significant improvements in blood pressure and overall cardiovascular health.

These comprehensive lifestyle modifications are essential for managing hypertension and improving long-term health outcomes.

Chapter 4: Medications for Hypertension

4.1 Antihypertensive Drug Classes

4.1.1 Diuretics

Diuretics, often referred to as "water pills," help reduce blood pressure by promoting the excretion of sodium and water from the body, thereby reducing blood volume.

- **Thiazide Diuretics**: Examples include hydrochlorothiazide and chlorthalidone.
- **Loop Diuretics**: Examples include furosemide and bumetanide.
- **Potassium-Sparing Diuretics**: Examples include spironolactone and amiloride.

4.1.2 ACE Inhibitors (Angiotensin-Converting Enzyme Inhibitors)

ACE inhibitors lower blood pressure by inhibiting the enzyme that converts angiotensin I to angiotensin II, a potent vasoconstrictor.

- **Examples**: Lisinopril, enalapril, and ramipril.

4.1.3 Angiotensin II Receptor Blockers (ARBs)

ARBs block the action of angiotensin II on its receptors, leading to vasodilation and reduced blood pressure.

- **Examples**: Losartan, valsartan, and irbesartan.

4.1.4 Calcium Channel Blockers

These medications prevent calcium from entering the cells of the heart and blood vessel walls, resulting in relaxed blood vessels and lower blood pressure.

- **Dihydropyridines**: Examples include amlodipine and nifedipine.
- **Non-Dihydropyridines**: Examples include verapamil and diltiazem.

4.1.5 Beta-Blockers

Beta-blockers reduce blood pressure by blocking the effects of adrenaline, leading to a slower heart rate and reduced force of heart contractions.

- **Examples**: Metoprolol, atenolol, and propranolol.

4.2 Mechanisms of Action

4.2.1 Diuretics

- **Pharmacodynamics**: Diuretics act on the kidneys to increase sodium and water excretion. This reduces blood volume and peripheral resistance.
- **Pharmacokinetics**: Diuretics are absorbed in the gastrointestinal tract, metabolized minimally, and excreted primarily through the urine.

4.2.2 ACE Inhibitors

- **Pharmacodynamics**: ACE inhibitors inhibit the conversion of angiotensin I to angiotensin II, reducing vasoconstriction and aldosterone secretion, leading to vasodilation and decreased blood volume.
- **Pharmacokinetics**: These drugs are absorbed orally, metabolized in the liver, and excreted by the kidneys.

4.2.3 ARBs

- **Pharmacodynamics**: ARBs selectively block the binding of angiotensin II to its receptor, preventing vasoconstriction and aldosterone-mediated volume expansion.
- **Pharmacokinetics**: ARBs are absorbed orally, metabolized in the liver, and excreted in urine and feces.

4.2.4 Calcium Channel Blockers

- **Pharmacodynamics**: These drugs inhibit the influx of calcium ions into vascular smooth muscle and cardiac cells, leading to vasodilation and reduced cardiac contractility.
- **Pharmacokinetics**: They are absorbed in the gastrointestinal tract, metabolized by the liver, and excreted primarily through the urine.

4.2.5 Beta-Blockers

- **Pharmacodynamics:** Beta-blockers block β-adrenergic receptors, reducing heart rate, myocardial contractility, and renin release from the kidneys.
- **Pharmacokinetics:** They are absorbed orally, metabolized in the liver, and excreted via the urine and feces.

4.3 Side Effects and Management

4.3.1 Diuretics

- **Common Side Effects:** Dehydration, electrolyte imbalance (e.g., hypokalemia), dizziness, and increased urination.
- **Management Strategies:** Monitoring electrolytes, maintaining adequate hydration, and using potassium-sparing diuretics or potassium supplements when necessary.

4.3.2 ACE Inhibitors

- **Common Side Effects:** Cough, elevated blood potassium levels (hyperkalemia), low blood pressure (hypotension), and kidney dysfunction.
- **Management Strategies:** Monitoring kidney function and potassium levels and switching to ARBs if a persistent cough develops.

4.3.3 ARBs

- **Common Side Effects:** Dizziness, hyperkalemia, and renal impairment.
- **Management Strategies:** Regularly monitor blood pressure, kidney function, and potassium levels.

4.3.4 Calcium Channel Blockers

- **Common Side Effects:** Edema, constipation, dizziness, and headache.
- **Management Strategies:** Adjusting the dose, switching to another class of antihypertensive, and using combination therapy to reduce side effects.

4.3.5 Beta-Blockers

- **Common Side Effects:** Fatigue, cold extremities, depression, and bradycardia (slow heart rate).

- **Management Strategies**: Gradual dose adjustment, monitoring heart rate, and considering alternative medications if side effects are intolerable.

4.4 Combination Therapy

4.4.1 Rationale for Combination Therapy

Combination therapy, using two or more antihypertensive agents with different mechanisms of action, is often more effective in achieving target blood pressure levels than monotherapy. It can also reduce the likelihood of side effects by allowing lower doses of each medication.

4.4.2 Fixed-Dose Combinations

Fixed-dose combinations (FDCs) are formulations that combine two or more antihypertensive agents into a single pill. Advantages include:

- **Improved Adherence**: Simplifies the medication regimen, increasing the likelihood that patients will take their medications as prescribed.
- **Enhanced Efficacy**: Combining drugs with complementary mechanisms can provide synergistic effects, improving blood pressure control.

4.4.3 Examples of Effective Combinations

- **ACE Inhibitor + Diuretic**: Commonly used to enhance the blood pressure-lowering effects while minimizing side effects.
- **ARB + Calcium Channel Blocker**: Effective for patients who cannot tolerate ACE inhibitors.
- **Beta-Blocker + Diuretic**: Often used in patients with additional cardiovascular conditions such as heart failure.

Clinical trials have demonstrated the effectiveness of combination therapy in managing hypertension, particularly in patients who do not achieve target blood pressure with monotherapy.

These sections provide a comprehensive overview of the pharmacological management of hypertension, detailing the various classes of antihypertensive drugs, their mechanisms of action, potential side effects, and the benefits of combination therapy. This information equips patients and families with the knowledge to make informed decisions about hypertension treatment options.

Chapter 5: Monitoring Your Blood Pressure

5.1 Home Blood Pressure Monitoring

5.1.1 Guidelines for Home Blood Pressure Monitoring

Home blood pressure monitoring (HBPM) is a valuable tool for managing hypertension and provides more consistent readings than occasional measurements at the doctor's office. Here are the guidelines for effective HBPM:

- **Device Selection:** Choose an automatic, validated, and clinically tested blood pressure monitor with an upper arm cuff. Wrist and finger monitors are generally less accurate.
- **Proper Cuff Size:** Ensure the cuff fits properly; an ill-fitting cuff can lead to inaccurate readings. The cuff should cover 80% of the arm circumference.

5.1.2 Proper Technique for Home Blood Pressure Monitoring

To obtain accurate and reliable readings, follow these best practices:

- **Preparation:** Rest for at least 5 minutes before measuring. Avoid caffeine, smoking, and exercise for at least 30 minutes prior.
- **Positioning:** Sit in a chair with your feet flat on the floor and back supported. Place the cuff on a bare arm at heart level, resting the arm on a flat surface.
- **Measurement Process:** Take two or three readings at each session, one minute apart. Record all readings and use the average for more accurate assessment.

5.1.3 Interpreting Results

- **Normal Range:** A normal blood pressure reading is usually around 120/80 mmHg. Consistently higher readings may indicate hypertension.
- **Hypertension Criteria:** For home measurements, hypertension is generally defined as a systolic pressure of 135 mmHg or higher, or a diastolic pressure of 85 mmHg or higher.
- **Consultation:** Regularly review your readings with your healthcare provider to make informed decisions about your treatment plan.

5.2 Ambulatory Blood Pressure Monitoring

5.2.1 Advantages of Ambulatory Blood Pressure Monitoring

Ambulatory blood pressure monitoring (ABPM) provides a comprehensive assessment of blood pressure over a 24-hour period, capturing variations throughout the day and night. Benefits include:

- **Accurate Diagnosis:** Detects white-coat hypertension (elevated readings in a clinical setting but not at home) and masked hypertension (normal readings in a clinical setting but elevated at home).
- **Comprehensive Data:** Provides detailed information on blood pressure patterns, including nocturnal hypertension (elevated blood pressure at night), which is linked to higher cardiovascular risk.
- **Better Management:** Helps tailor antihypertensive treatment by identifying times of day when blood pressure is highest.

5.2.2 Indications for Ambulatory Blood Pressure Monitoring

ABPM is recommended in several scenarios:

- **Suspected White-Coat or Masked Hypertension:** To confirm the diagnosis.
- **Resistant Hypertension:** When blood pressure remains high despite treatment with three or more antihypertensive medications.
- **Variable Blood Pressure Readings:** When readings fluctuate significantly, making it difficult to establish a consistent pattern.

5.2.3 How to Use Ambulatory Blood Pressure Monitoring

- **Device Setup:** A portable blood pressure monitor is worn for 24 hours, typically on the non-dominant arm. The device takes readings at regular intervals, usually every 15-30 minutes during the day and every 30-60 minutes at night.
- **Daily Activities:** Patients are advised to maintain their usual activities but avoid heavy exercise and bathing while wearing the monitor.
- **Data Analysis:** After 24 hours, the data is downloaded and analyzed by the healthcare provider to identify patterns and trends in blood pressure.

5.3 Keeping a Blood Pressure Diary

5.3.1 Importance of a Blood Pressure Diary

Maintaining a blood pressure diary helps track trends over time, identify triggers that may cause blood pressure fluctuations, and provides valuable information for healthcare providers to adjust treatment plans effectively.

5.3.2 Tips for Effective Record-Keeping

- **Consistency:** Record blood pressure readings at the same times each day, preferably in the morning and evening.
- **Comprehensive Entries:** Include additional information such as the date, time, reading (systolic/diastolic), heart rate, medication intake, diet, physical activity, stress levels, and any symptoms experienced.
- **Pattern Identification:** Review the diary regularly to identify patterns or triggers that may affect blood pressure, such as diet, physical activity, stress, or medication adherence.
- **Communication:** Share the diary with your healthcare provider during visits to provide a detailed picture of your blood pressure management and aid in making informed treatment decisions.

5.3.3 Example of a Blood Pressure Diary Entry

Date: 2024-06-14
Time: 8:00 AM
Blood Pressure: 130/85 mmHg
Heart Rate: 75 bpm
Medications: Lisinopril 10 mg
Diet: Breakfast - oatmeal with fruit
Physical Activity: 30-minute walk
Stress Levels: Low
Symptoms: None

By following these guidelines and best practices for home blood pressure monitoring, using ambulatory blood pressure monitoring when necessary, and maintaining a detailed blood pressure diary, patients and families can effectively manage hypertension and work collaboratively with healthcare providers to achieve better health outcomes.

Chapter 6: Support for Patients and Families

6.1 Role of Family and Caregivers

6.1.1 Emotional Support

Family members and caregivers play a vital role in providing emotional support to patients with hypertension. Their encouragement can significantly impact the patient's ability to cope with the condition and adhere to treatment plans. Emotional support involves:

- **Listening and Empathy:** Offering a sympathetic ear and understanding the patient's concerns and fears.
- **Motivation:** Encouraging the patient to stay committed to lifestyle changes and treatment plans.
- **Stress Reduction:** Identify and reduce sources of stress in the patient's life, which can positively affect blood pressure.

6.1.2 Assistance with Medication Adherence

Caregivers can help ensure that patients take their medications as prescribed, which is crucial for effective hypertension management. This can include:

- **Organizing Medication:** Using pill organizers to sort medications by day and time.
- **Setting Reminders:** Setting alarms or using mobile apps to remind patients to take their medications.
- **Monitoring Side Effects:** Keeping track of any side effects and communicating with healthcare providers to adjust treatment if necessary.

6.1.3 Support with Lifestyle Changes

Adopting and maintaining healthy lifestyle changes is easier with the support of family members and caregivers. This can involve:

- **Healthy Eating:** Preparing and sharing healthy meals that adhere to dietary recommendations, such as the DASH diet.
- **Exercise:** Participating in physical activities together to motivate the patient and make exercise more enjoyable.
- **Avoiding Triggers:** Helping the patient avoid lifestyle factors that can worsen hypertension, such as smoking and excessive alcohol consumption.

6.2 Patient Education

6.2.1 Understanding Hypertension

Educating patients about hypertension is fundamental for effective management. Key topics include:

- **What is Hypertension**: Explain the condition, causes, and potential complications.
- **Risk Factors**: Identifying personal risk factors, such as family history, lifestyle habits, and comorbid conditions.

6.2.2 Importance of Health Literacy

Health literacy is crucial for patients to understand and manage their condition effectively. Strategies for improving health literacy include:

- **Simplified Information**: Providing information in a clear, concise manner, avoiding medical jargon.
- **Educational Materials**: Using brochures, videos, and websites designed for patients with varying levels of health literacy.
- **Interactive Education**: Engaging patients through interactive workshops, group sessions, and one-on-one counseling.

6.2.3 Self-Management Skills

Teaching patient self-management skills empowers them to take control of their health. This involves:

- **Monitoring Blood Pressure**: Instruct patients to correctly measure their blood pressure at home.
- **Recognizing Symptoms**: Educating patients on symptoms of high blood pressure and when to seek medical help.
- **Adherence to Treatment**: Emphasize taking medications as prescribed, and attending regular follow-up appointments is important.

6.3 Support Groups and Resources

6.3.1 Support Groups

Support groups provide a platform for patients and families to share experiences, gain emotional support, and learn from others facing similar challenges. Benefits include:

- **Peer Support:** Connecting with others who understand the challenges of managing hypertension.
- **Shared Knowledge:** Learning about effective strategies and resources from group members.

6.3.2 Counseling Services

Professional counseling services can help patients and families cope with the emotional and psychological aspects of hypertension. This includes:

- **Stress Management:** Learn techniques to manage stress, which can positively impact blood pressure.
- **Behavioral Therapy:** Addressing behaviors that contribute to hypertension, such as poor diet and lack of exercise.

6.3.3 Online Resources

The Internet offers a wealth of resources for patients and families, including:

- **Educational Websites:** Trusted sources like the American Heart Association (AHA) and World Health Organization (WHO) provide comprehensive information on hypertension.
- **Mobile Apps:** Apps designed for hypertension management can help track blood pressure readings, medication adherence, and lifestyle changes.
- **Forums and Social Media:** Online communities and forums where patients can connect, ask questions, and share experiences.

Example Resources

- **American Heart Association:** www.heart.org - Offers extensive resources on hypertension, including educational materials, healthy living tips, and support group information.
- **World Health Organization:** www.who.int - Provides global health information and guidelines on hypertension.
- **MyFitnessPal:** www.myfitnesspal.com - A mobile app for tracking diet and exercise, helpful for weight management and lifestyle changes.

By leveraging the support of family and caregivers, educating patients, and utilizing available resources, individuals with hypertension can achieve better health outcomes and improve their quality of life.

Chapter 7: Navigating Hypertension in Special Situations

7.1 Hypertension in Pregnancy

7.1.1 Overview and Risks

Hypertension in pregnancy is a significant concern, as it poses risks to both the mother and the developing fetus. Types of hypertensive disorders in pregnancy include chronic hypertension, gestational hypertension, preeclampsia, and eclampsia.

Risks to the Mother:

- **Preeclampsia:** Characterized by high blood pressure and signs of damage to another organ system, often the kidneys. It can lead to serious complications like placental abruption, organ damage, and eclampsia.
- **Eclampsia:** The onset of seizures in a woman with preeclampsia, a medical emergency requiring immediate intervention.
- **Chronic Hypertension:** Increases the risk of developing preeclampsia and other complications.

Risks to the Baby:

- **Intrauterine Growth Restriction (IUGR):** High blood pressure can reduce blood flow to the placenta, affecting fetal growth.
- **Preterm Birth:** Hypertension increases the risk of preterm delivery, which can lead to complications associated with prematurity.
- **Stillbirth:** Severe hypertensive disorders can increase the risk of fetal death.

7.1.2 Management Strategies

Management of hypertension during pregnancy involves careful monitoring and treatment to minimize risks to both the mother and the baby.

Monitoring:

- **Frequent Prenatal Visits:** Regular check-ups to monitor blood pressure, urine protein levels, and fetal growth.
- **Fetal Monitoring:** Ultrasounds and non-stress tests to assess fetal well-being.

Treatment Options:

- **Lifestyle Modifications:** Dietary changes, reduced salt intake, and regular physical activity as advised by a healthcare provider.
- **Medications:** Antihypertensive medications that are safe for use during pregnancy, such as methyldopa, labetalol, and nifedipine. ACE inhibitors and angiotensin II receptor blockers are generally avoided due to potential harm to the fetus.
- **Delivery Planning:** In cases of severe preeclampsia or eclampsia, early delivery may be necessary to protect the health of the mother and baby.

7.2 Hypertension in Older Adults

7.2.1 Challenges and Considerations

Managing hypertension in older adults presents unique challenges due to age-related physiological changes, the presence of comorbid conditions, and the increased likelihood of polypharmacy.

Age-Related Changes:

- **Arterial Stiffness:** Aging leads to decreased elasticity of the arteries, contributing to higher systolic blood pressure.
- **Renal Function Decline:** Reduced kidney function can affect blood pressure regulation and response to medications.

Comorbid Conditions:

- **Diabetes:** Common in older adults and complicates hypertension management.
- **Cardiovascular Disease:** Prevalent in the elderly, requiring careful management of blood pressure to prevent further complications.

7.2.2 Polypharmacy

Older adults often take multiple medications for various health issues, increasing the risk of drug interactions and side effects.

Strategies to Manage Polypharmacy:

- **Medication Review:** Review all medications regularly by healthcare providers to minimize unnecessary prescriptions and reduce the risk of adverse interactions.
- **Simplified Regimens:** Using combination medications when appropriate to reduce pill burden.

7.2.3 Treatment Approaches

- **Lifestyle Modifications:** Emphasizing a heart-healthy diet, regular physical activity, and weight management.
- **Medication Adjustments:** Tailoring antihypertensive therapy to the individual's health status and monitor frequently for side effects.
- **Blood Pressure Targets:** Adjusting treatment goals to balance the benefits of lowering blood pressure against the risks of potential side effects such as falls or orthostatic hypotension.

7.3 Pediatric Hypertension

7.3.1 Overview

Hypertension in children and adolescents is increasingly recognized as a significant health issue, often associated with obesity and other lifestyle factors. Early diagnosis and management are crucial to prevent long-term health complications.

7.3.2 Diagnosis

Diagnosing hypertension in children requires careful measurement and interpretation of blood pressure values based on age, sex, and height percentiles.

Screening and Diagnosis:

- **Routine Check-ups:** Regular blood pressure measurements during pediatric visits.
- **Confirmatory Testing:** Ambulatory blood pressure monitoring to confirm hypertension and rule out white-coat hypertension.

7.3.3 Causes and Risk Factors

- **Primary Hypertension:** More common in adolescents and often linked to obesity, family history, and lifestyle factors.
- **Secondary Hypertension:** More prevalent in younger children, caused by underlying conditions such as kidney disease, endocrine disorders, or congenital heart defects.

7.3.4 Management Strategies

Lifestyle Modifications:

- **Dietary Changes:** Emphasizing a balanced diet rich in fruits, vegetables, whole grains, and low-fat dairy products, while reducing salt and sugar intake.
- **Physical Activity:** Encouraging regular exercise, with at least 60 minutes of moderate-to-vigorous physical activity daily.

Medication:

- **Pharmacologic Treatment:** Antihypertensive medications may be necessary for children with persistent hypertension or underlying health conditions. The choice of medications and dosage is carefully tailored to the child's needs and monitored closely.

7.3.5 Long-Term Follow-Up

- **Regular Monitoring:** Continue to assess blood pressure, growth, and development.
- **Education:** Teaching children and their families the importance of adherence to lifestyle changes and treatment plans to ensure long-term health benefits.

By addressing these special situations with tailored approaches, healthcare providers can effectively manage hypertension in diverse populations, improving outcomes for pregnant women, older adults, and children.

Chapter 8: Resources for Managing Hypertension

8.1 Technology and Mobile Apps

8.1.1 The Role of Technology in Hypertension Management

Technology has revolutionized the management of hypertension, offering tools that help patients monitor their condition, adhere to treatment plans, and make informed decisions about their health.

Benefits of Technology:

- **Convenience:** Easy-to-use apps and devices facilitate regular monitoring and record-keeping.
- **Real-Time Data:** Instant access to data allows for timely adjustments in treatment and lifestyle.
- **Motivation:** Interactive features and reminders help keep patients engaged and compliant.

8.1.2 Mobile Apps for Hypertension Management

Mobile apps offer a range of functionalities, from tracking blood pressure readings to providing educational content and medication reminders.

Popular and Effective Apps:

- **MyFitnessPal:** Tracks diet and exercise, helping users adhere to heart-healthy lifestyle changes.
- **Blood Pressure Companion:** Allows users to record and monitor blood pressure readings, set reminders for medication, and visualize trends.
- **Heart Habit:** Integrates with wearable devices to monitor blood pressure and offers personalized insights and coaching.
- **Omron Connect:** Syncs with Omron blood pressure monitors, providing a seamless way to track and manage readings.

8.1.3 Wearable Devices

Wearable technology, such as smartwatches and fitness trackers, can continuously monitor vital signs and provide valuable data for managing hypertension.

Popular Wearable Devices:

- **Apple Watch:** Features an ECG app that will track heart rate and physical activity, helping users maintain a healthy lifestyle.

- **Fitbit Charge:** Monitors heart rate, sleep patterns, and physical activity, providing insights into overall health and fitness.
- **Withings BPM Core:** A blood pressure monitor that can detect atrial fibrillation and record heart sounds, offering comprehensive cardiovascular health tracking.

8.2 Educational Materials

8.2.1 Reliable Sources of Information

Access to accurate and reliable educational materials is crucial for patients and their families to understand and manage hypertension effectively.

Books:

- **"The DASH Diet Action Plan" by Marla Heller:** A comprehensive guide to the DASH diet, providing practical advice on implementing this heart-healthy eating plan.
- **"Hypertension and You: Old Drugs, New Drugs, and the Right Drugs for Your High Blood Pressure" by Samuel J. Mann:** Offers insights into medication management and lifestyle changes for controlling hypertension.

Websites:

- **American Heart Association (AHA):** www.heart.org - Provides extensive information on hypertension, including prevention, management, and treatment options.
- **World Health Organization (WHO):** www.who.int - Offers global guidelines and information on hypertension and cardiovascular health.
- **National Heart, Lung, and Blood Institute (NHLBI):** www.nhlbi.nih.gov - Features educational resources on high blood pressure, including research findings and treatment recommendations.

8.2.2 Educational Videos

Videos can be an engaging way to learn about hypertension and its management. Many reputable health organizations and experts offer video content that explains various aspects of hypertension in an easy-to-understand format.

Recommended Video Resources:

- **YouTube Channels:**
    - **American Heart Association:** Provides videos on hypertension management, healthy living, and patient stories.
    - **Mayo Clinic:** Offers educational videos on hypertension, including lifestyle tips, treatment options, and expert interviews.
- **Online Courses and Webinars:** Coursera, Khan Academy, and other websites offer health-related courses that include modules on hypertension and cardiovascular health.

8.3 Community Resources

8.3.1 Community Programs and Services

Community resources can provide additional support for individuals managing hypertension, offering programs and services that promote healthy living and disease management.

Local Health Departments:

- **Health Education Programs:** Local health departments often offer classes and workshops on hypertension, covering topics such as diet, exercise, and medication management.
- **Screening Services:** Many health departments provide free or low-cost blood pressure screening services to help individuals monitor their condition.

8.3.2 Support Groups

Support groups can provide a sense of community and shared experience, helping individuals manage hypertension more effectively.

Benefits of Support Groups:

- **Emotional Support:** Connecting with others who face similar challenges can reduce feelings of isolation and stress.
- **Shared Knowledge:** Group members can share tips, resources, and experiences, providing practical advice and support.

8.3.3 Fitness and Wellness Programs

Local gyms, community centers, and wellness programs often offer classes and activities that support heart health and hypertension management.

Examples of Programs:

- **Exercise Classes:** Programs like walking clubs, yoga classes, and water aerobics can help individuals stay active and manage blood pressure.
- **Nutrition Workshops:** Many community centers offer cooking classes and nutrition workshops that teach participants how to prepare heart-healthy meals.

8.3.4 Online Communities and Forums

Online communities and forums can provide a platform for individuals to ask questions, share experiences, and receive support from a broader community.

Popular Online Communities:

- **Reddit:** Subreddits like r/Hypertension offer a space for individuals to discuss their experiences and seek advice.
- **HealthUnlocked:** A social network for health that includes communities focused on hypertension and cardiovascular health.

By utilizing these various resources, patients and their families can gain the knowledge, support, and tools for managing hypertension and improving overall health.

Chapter 9: Planning for the Future

9.1 Setting Goals

9.1.1 Importance of Goal Setting

Setting realistic and achievable goals is crucial for effective long-term management of hypertension. Goals provide a clear direction and motivation, helping patients stay focused and committed to their treatment plans.

9.1.2 Strategies for Goal Setting

SMART Goals

Utilizing the SMART criteria ensures that goals are Specific, Measurable, Achievable, Relevant, and Time-bound. This approach helps in creating clear and actionable objectives.

- **Specific:** Clearly define what you want to achieve. For example, "Reduce systolic blood pressure by 10 mmHg."
- **Measurable:** Ensure that the goal can be quantified. For example, "Track blood pressure readings daily."
- **Achievable:** Set goals that are realistic given your current health status and resources. For example, "Incorporate 30 minutes of moderate exercise into daily routine."
- **Relevant:** Align goals with overall health objectives. For example, "Follow a low-sodium diet to help lower blood pressure."
- **Time-bound:** Set a deadline for achieving the goal. For example, "Achieve target blood pressure within six months."

Incremental Goals

Breaking down larger goals into smaller, manageable steps can make the process less overwhelming and more achievable. For example, start with a goal of reducing sodium intake by 500 mg per day and gradually decrease further.

9.1.3 Monitoring Progress

Regularly tracking progress towards goals helps in maintaining motivation and making necessary adjustments. Tools such as blood pressure diaries, mobile apps, and regular consultations with healthcare providers can assist in this process.

9.2 Regular Check-Ups

9.2.1 Importance of Medical Check-Ups

Regular check-ups with healthcare providers are essential for effective hypertension management. These visits provide an opportunity to monitor blood pressure, assess the effectiveness of treatment plans, and make necessary adjustments.

9.2.2 Frequency of Check-Ups

The frequency of check-ups can vary depending on the individual's health status, the severity of hypertension, and any underlying health conditions. Typically, patients with well-controlled hypertension might see their doctor every 3-6 months, while those with uncontrolled hypertension may require more frequent visits.

9.2.3 Communication with Healthcare Providers

Open and ongoing communication with healthcare providers is vital. Patients should feel comfortable discussing their concerns, reporting any side effects of medications, and seeking advice on lifestyle modifications. Effective communication ensures that treatment plans are tailored to the patient's needs and preferences.

9.2.4 Comprehensive Health Assessments

Regular check-ups should include comprehensive health assessments beyond blood pressure measurement. This includes monitoring kidney function, assessing cardiovascular risk, and screening for related conditions such as diabetes and dyslipidemia.

9.3 Long-Term Management

9.3.1 Adapting to Changes in Health Status

Over time, changes in health status, such as aging, the development of new health conditions, or changes in lifestyle, may necessitate adjustments in hypertension management strategies.

Aging and Hypertension

As patients age, physiological changes can impact blood pressure regulation and the response to medications. Regular reassessment of treatment plans is crucial to address these changes.

Comorbid Conditions

The presence of other health conditions, such as diabetes, kidney disease, or cardiovascular disease, can complicate hypertension management. Integrated care approaches that address all aspects of a patient's health are essential for effective long-term management.

9.3.2 Advancing Medical Knowledge

Staying informed about the latest advancements in medical knowledge and treatment options is important for both patients and healthcare providers. This can include new medications, innovative treatment approaches, and updated clinical guidelines.

Continuing Education

Patients should be encouraged to engage in continuous learning about hypertension and its management. This can be facilitated through resources such as educational materials, support groups, and health literacy programs.

Research and Clinical Trials

Participation in clinical trials can provide access to cutting-edge treatments and contribute to the advancement of medical knowledge. Patients should discuss potential opportunities with their healthcare providers.

9.3.3 Maintaining Lifestyle Changes

Sustaining healthy lifestyle changes over the long term is critical for maintaining blood pressure control. This includes adhering to dietary recommendations, maintaining regular physical activity, managing stress, and avoiding tobacco and excessive alcohol use.

Behavioral Strategies

Employing behavioral strategies such as setting reminders, seeking social support, and using motivational tools can help maintain lifestyle changes.

Support Systems

Building a strong support system, including family, friends, healthcare providers, and community resources, can provide ongoing encouragement and assistance.

9.3.4 Monitoring and Adjusting Treatment Plans

Continuous monitoring and periodic reassessment of treatment plans are necessary to ensure their effectiveness. This involves:

- **Regular Blood Pressure Monitoring**: Keeping track of blood pressure readings to identify trends and make timely adjustments.
- **Medication Review**: Periodically reviewing medications to ensure they are effective and adjusting dosages or switching medications as needed.
- **Lifestyle Assessment**: Evaluating adherence to lifestyle modifications and making necessary changes to enhance their impact.

By setting realistic goals, maintaining regular check-ups, and adopting a proactive approach to long-term management, patients can effectively navigate the complexities of hypertension and improve their overall health outcomes.

Chapter 10: Conclusion

10.1 Summary of Key Points

Understanding Hypertension

- **Definition and Epidemiology**: Hypertension, or high blood pressure, is a chronic condition with widespread prevalence globally. It can be categorized into primary and secondary hypertension, with various risk factors affecting different demographic groups.
- **Pathophysiology**: Hypertension involves complex mechanisms including the autonomic nervous system, renal function, and the renin-angiotensin-aldosterone system, influenced by genetic, environmental, and behavioral factors.
- **Complications**: Chronic hypertension can lead to severe complications like heart disease, stroke, kidney failure, and vision loss, underscoring the importance of effective management.

Diagnosing Hypertension

- **Blood Pressure Measurement Techniques**: Accurate measurement methods, including office, home, and ambulatory monitoring, are crucial for proper diagnosis.
- **Diagnostic Criteria**: Defined by major health organizations, these criteria help in identifying hypertension and its severity.
- **Secondary Hypertension Screening**: Identifying underlying causes through diagnostic tests ensures appropriate treatment.

Managing Hypertension Through Lifestyle Modifications

- **Dietary Interventions**: The DASH diet, reducing sodium intake, and ensuring adequate potassium, magnesium, and calcium are vital dietary strategies.
- **Physical Activity**: Regular exercise, including aerobic, resistance, and flexibility exercises, significantly helps manage blood pressure.
- **Weight Management**: Addressing obesity through diet, exercise, and behavioral changes is essential for controlling hypertension.
- **Stress Management**: Techniques like mindfulness, meditation, and cognitive-behavioral therapy effectively reduce stress and blood pressure.
- **Alcohol and Tobacco Use**: Reducing or eliminating alcohol and tobacco use is critical for managing hypertension.

Medications for Hypertension

- **Antihypertensive Drug Classes**: Various classes, including diuretics, ACE inhibitors, ARBs, calcium channel blockers, and beta-blockers, offer different mechanisms for lowering blood pressure.

- **Mechanisms of Action:** Understanding pharmacodynamics and pharmacokinetics helps in selecting appropriate medications.
- **Side Effects and Management:** Awareness of potential side effects and strategies for managing them aids in adherence and effectiveness.
- **Combination Therapy:** Combining medications can enhance efficacy and reduce side effects, improving overall management.

Monitoring Your Blood Pressure

- **Home Blood Pressure Monitoring:** Best practices for home monitoring, including device selection and proper technique, help maintain accurate records.
- **Ambulatory Blood Pressure Monitoring:** This method provides a comprehensive assessment over 24 hours, aiding in more accurate diagnosis and management.
- **Keeping a Blood Pressure Diary:** Maintaining a diary helps track trends and informs healthcare decisions.

Support for Patients and Families

- **Role of Family and Caregivers:** Family members and caregivers provide crucial emotional support and assistance with adherence to treatment plans.
- **Patient Education:** Effective education strategies enhance health literacy and empower patients to manage their condition.
- **Support Groups and Resources:** Access to support groups, counseling services, and online resources provides additional help for patients and families.

Navigating Hypertension in Special Situations

- **Hypertension in Pregnancy:** Management strategies to minimize risks to mother and baby, including monitoring and safe medications.
- **Hypertension in Older Adults:** Addressing age-related changes and comorbidities, with a focus on polypharmacy and individualized treatment.
- **Pediatric Hypertension:** Diagnosis and management tailored to children and adolescents, considering unique factors and treatment approaches.

Resources for Managing Hypertension

- **Technology and Mobile Apps:** Tools like mobile apps and wearable devices assist in monitoring and managing hypertension.
- **Educational Materials:** Reliable books, websites, and videos provide valuable information on hypertension.
- **Community Resources:** Local programs and services offer support and resources for managing hypertension.

Planning for the Future

- **Setting Goals:** Strategies for setting realistic, achievable goals to maintain blood pressure control.
- **Regular Check-Ups:** The importance of ongoing medical check-ups and communication with healthcare providers.
- **Long-Term Management:** Approaches for sustaining blood pressure control, adapting to health changes, and keeping up with advancing medical knowledge.

10.2 Future Directions

Emerging Treatments

Research continues to explore new treatments for hypertension, including novel medications, gene therapy, and innovative technologies. Advances in pharmacology aim to develop drugs with fewer side effects and more targeted actions.

Personalized Medicine

The future of hypertension management lies in personalized medicine, which tailors treatment to the individual based on genetic, environmental, and lifestyle factors. Personalized approaches can enhance the effectiveness of treatments and minimize adverse effects.

Technological Innovations

The integration of artificial intelligence and machine learning into healthcare holds promise for hypertension management. Predictive analytics, personalized recommendations, and advanced monitoring systems can improve patient outcomes.

Public Health Initiatives

Ongoing public health efforts aim to reduce the incidence of hypertension through community education, policy changes, and preventive measures. These initiatives focus on promoting healthy lifestyles and improving access to healthcare.

10.3 Final Thoughts

Significance of Patient and Family Engagement

Effective management of hypertension requires active engagement from both patients and their families. Education, support, and involvement in the treatment process are key to achieving and maintaining blood pressure control.

Call to Action

Continued education and support for patients, families, and healthcare providers are essential for combating hypertension. Emphasizing the importance of lifestyle changes, regular monitoring, and adherence to treatment plans can lead to better health outcomes.

By integrating comprehensive management strategies and leveraging emerging technologies and treatments, we can improve the lives of those affected by hypertension and move towards a future with better prevention and control of this widespread condition.

Thank you for exploring *Navigating Hypertension*! If you found this book valuable, consider sharing it with friends, family, or colleagues who might benefit from the information. Together, we can empower more people to take control of their health.

And remember, knowledge shared is knowledge multiplied!

References by Chapter

Chapter 1: Understanding Hypertension

1. **American Heart Association (AHA).** "Understanding Blood Pressure Readings." Available at: https://www.heart.org/en/health-topics/high-blood-pressure/understanding-blood-pressure-readings
2. **World Health Organization (WHO).** "Hypertension." Available at: https://www.who.int/news-room/fact-sheets/detail/hypertension
3. **Carretero, O. A., & Oparil, S.** (2000). "Essential Hypertension: Part I: Definition and Etiology." Circulation, 101(3), 329-335. doi:10.1161/01.CIR.101.3.329

Chapter 2: Diagnosing Hypertension

4. **Pickering, T. G., et al.** (2005). "Recommendations for Blood Pressure Measurement in Humans and Experimental Animals Part 1: Blood Pressure Measurement in Humans." Hypertension, 45(1), 142-161. doi:10.1161/01.HYP.0000150859.47929.8e
5. **National Institute for Health and Care Excellence (NICE).** "Hypertension in Adults: Diagnosis and Management." Available at: https://www.nice.org.uk/guidance/ng136
6. **Messerli, F. H., Williams, B., & Ritz, E.** (2007). "Essential Hypertension." The Lancet, 370(9587), 591-603. doi:10.1016/S0140-6736(07)61299-9

Chapter 3: Managing Hypertension Through Lifestyle Modifications

7. **Sacks, F. M., et al.** (2001). "Effects on Blood Pressure of Reduced Dietary Sodium and the Dietary Approaches to Stop Hypertension (DASH) Diet." New England Journal of Medicine, 344(1), 3-10. doi:10.1056/NEJM200101043440101
8. **Pescatello, L. S., et al.** (2004). "Exercise and Hypertension." Medicine & Science in Sports & Exercise, 36(3), 533-553. doi:10.1249/01.MSS.0000115224.88514.3A
9. **American College of Cardiology (ACC).** "Managing Hypertension with Lifestyle Modifications." Available at: https://www.acc.org/latest-in-cardiology/articles/2019/05/09/12/42/managing-hypertension-with-lifestyle-modifications

Chapter 4: Medications for Hypertension

10. **James, P. A., et al.** (2014). "2014 Evidence-Based Guideline for the Management of High Blood Pressure in Adults." JAMA, 311(5), 507-520. doi:10.1001/jama.2013.284427
11. **Chobanian, A. V., et al.** (2003). "Seventh Report of the Joint National Committee on Prevention, Detection, Evaluation, and Treatment of High Blood Pressure." Hypertension, 42(6), 1206-1252. doi:10.1161/01.HYP.0000107251.49515.c2
12. **Weber, M. A., et al.** (2014). "Clinical Practice Guidelines for the Management of Hypertension in the Community." Journal of Clinical Hypertension, 16(1), 14-26. doi:10.1111/jch.12237

Chapter 5: Monitoring Your Blood Pressure

13. **O'Brien, E., et al.** (2003). "European Society of Hypertension Recommendations for Conventional, Ambulatory, and Home Blood Pressure Measurement." Journal of Hypertension, 21(5), 821-848. doi:10.1097/01.hjh.0000059016.82022.9a
14. **Parati, G., et al.** (2008). "Clinical Relevance of Day-by-Day Blood Pressure and Hypertension Variability." Hypertension, 52(4), 632-639. doi:10.1161/HYPERTENSIONAHA.107.105080
15. **Stergiou, G. S., et al.** (2014). "Home Blood Pressure Monitoring: Primary Care Physician and Patient Perspectives." The Journal of Clinical Hypertension, 16(5), 336-341. doi:10.1111/jch.12297

Chapter 6: Support for Patients and Families

16. **American Heart Association (AHA).** "Support Network for Patients with High Blood Pressure." Available at: https://supportnetwork.heart.org/
17. **Bodenheimer, T., et al.** (2002). "Patient Self-management of Chronic Disease in Primary Care." JAMA, 288(19), 2469-2475. doi:10.1001/jama.288.19.2469
18. **Lorig, K. R., et al.** (2001). "Chronic Disease Self-Management Program: 2-Year Health Status and Health Care Utilization Outcomes." Medical Care, 39(11), 1217-1223. doi:10.1097/00005650-200111000-00008

Chapter 7: Navigating Hypertension in Special Situations

19. **American College of Obstetricians and Gynecologists (ACOG).** "Hypertension in Pregnancy." Available at: https://www.acog.org/clinical/clinical-guidance/task-force-and-work-group-reports/articles/2013/11/hypertension-in-pregnancy
20. **Aronow, W. S., & Fleg, J. L.** (2011). "Hypertension in the Elderly." In *Hypertension: A Companion to Braunwald's Heart Disease* (pp. 318-327). Elsevier.
21. **Flynn, J. T., et al.** (2017). "Clinical Practice Guideline for Screening and Management of High Blood Pressure in Children and Adolescents." Pediatrics, 140(3), e20171904. doi:10.1542/peds.2017-1904

Chapter 8: Resources for Managing Hypertension

22. **Free, C., et al.** (2013). "The Effectiveness of Mobile-Health Technology-Based Health Behaviour Change or Disease Management Interventions for Health Care Consumers: A Systematic Review." PLOS Medicine, 10(1), e1001362. doi:10.1371/journal.pmed.1001362
23. **American Heart Association (AHA).** "Educational Materials on Hypertension." Available at: https://www.heart.org/en/health-topics/high-blood-pressure
24. **Centers for Disease Control and Prevention (CDC).** "High Blood Pressure Tools and Resources." Available at: https://www.cdc.gov/bloodpressure/tools.htm

Chapter 9: Planning for the Future

25. **Lewington, S., et al.** (2002). "Age-Specific Relevance of Usual Blood Pressure to Vascular Mortality: A Meta-analysis of Individual Data for One Million Adults in 61 Prospective Studies." The Lancet, 360(9349), 1903-1913. doi:10.1016/S0140-6736(02)11911-8
26. **Whelton, P. K., et al.** (2017). "2017 ACC/AHA/AAPA/ABC/ACPM/AGS/APhA/ASH/ASPC/NMA/PCNA Guideline for the Prevention, Detection, Evaluation, and Management of High Blood Pressure in Adults." Hypertension, 71(6), e13-e115. doi:10.1161/HYP.0000000000000065
27. **Centers for Disease Control and Prevention (CDC).** "Managing Blood Pressure: A Lifetime Commitment." Available at: https://www.cdc.gov/bloodpressure/management.htm

www.ingramcontent.com/pod-product-compliance
Lightning Source LLC
LaVergne TN
LVHW081549070526
838199LV00061B/4254